YOGA
FOR
STIFF BIRDS

MARION DEUCHARS

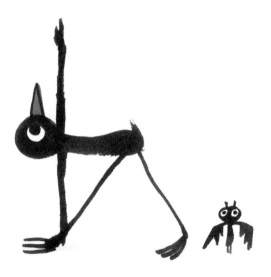

🦢 Skittledog

THIS BOOK IS INTENDED TO HELP THOSE
WHO ARE NEW TO YOGA AND INSPIRE
OTHERS WHO HAVE ALREADY STARTED
THEIR YOGA JOURNEY.

IT'S A BOOK FOR BIRDS OF ALL FEATHERS.

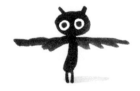

✳ CONSULT A DOCTOR BEFORE BEGINNING
ANY NEW EXERCISE REGIME.

INTRODUCTION

YOGA IS A PHILOSOPHY THAT FIRST DEVELOPED IN INDIA AROUND 2500 YEARS AGO, THOUGH THE EXACT DATE IS UNKNOWN. THE WORD YOGA COMES FROM THE SANSKRIT WORD 'YUT', MEANING 'TO JOIN' AND TO CONCENTRATE ONE'S ATTENTION.

MANY PEOPLE NOW ASSOCIATE YOGA WITH PHYSICAL POSES ('ASANA' IN SANSKRIT), WHICH CAN BE PRACTISED TO SLOW YOU DOWN, HELP YOU TO BREATHE BETTER, RELIEVE STRESS, BECOME FITTER OR MORE FLEXIBLE, INCREASE SEROTONIN LEVELS AND CULTIVATE A SENSE OF WELL-BEING. IT'S NEVER TOO LATE TO START LEARNING AND BECOME FAMILIAR WITH A FEW ASANAS.

YOU CAN DO YOGA AT HOME, IN A CLASS OR ONLINE. ALWAYS START SLOWLY AND NEVER PUSH YOUR BODY TO A PLACE THAT FEELS PAINFUL. HOLD EACH POSE FOR A FEW BREATHS TO ALLOW BODY, BREATH AND MIND TO SETTLE. AND ALWAYS COME OUT CALMLY IF YOU ARE UNCOMFORTABLE.

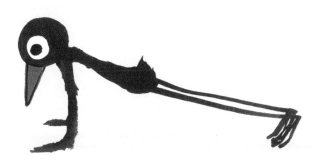

WHERE to START?

START WITH A COMFORTABLE
SEATED POSE. IT IS ONE
THAT IS MOST ASSOCIATED
WITH YOGA PRACTICE AND
SO A GOOD PLACE TO START.

EASY/COMFORTABLE
Sukhasana

SIT CROSS- LEGGED.
USE A BLOCK OR
ROLLED-UP TOWEL IF
NEEDED UNDER YOUR
BOTTOM. BROADEN
SHOULDERS, LENGTHEN
NECK. HANDS ON LAP.

DEEP,
SLOW
BREATHS

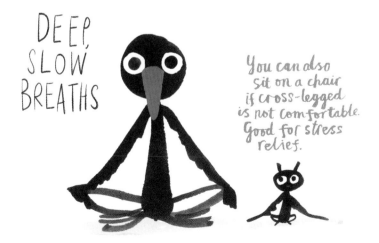

You can also
sit on a chair
if cross-legged
is not comfortable.
Good for stress
relief.

YOGA FLOW TO ENERGISE THE BODY AND WAKE UP SPINE.
REPEAT 3 TIMES.

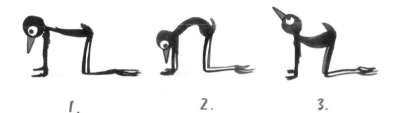

1.   2.   3.

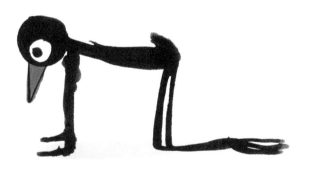

1. TABLE TOP

Bharmanasana

BEGIN ON ALL FOURS, HIPS
OVER KNEES, SHOULDERS
OVER WRISTS. KNEES
HIP-DISTANCE APART.

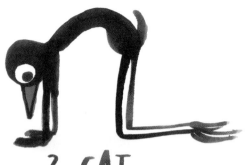

2. <u>CAT</u>

Marjariasana

EXHALE AS YOU DRAW TAILBONE DOWN, ROUND YOUR SPINE, AND RELAX THE NECK. DRAW YOUR BELLY IN AND UP.

Deep stretch

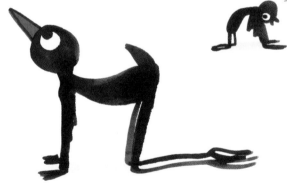

3. <u>COW</u>

Bitilasana

INHALE AS YOU ARCH YOUR BACK, RELAX TUMMY, DRAW SHOULDERS AWAY FROM EARS. EXTEND NECK UP.

PLANK

Kumbhakasana

START BY LYING FACE
DOWN. BEND ELBOWS
AND PLACE HANDS FLAT
UNDER SHOULDERS. TUCK
TOES UNDER. KEEPING
TUMMY FIRM, LIFT BODY
AND SHIFT WEIGHT TO
HANDS AND TOES. IMAGINE
A DIAGONAL LINE EXTENDING
FROM TOES TO FOREHEAD
AND BEYOND.

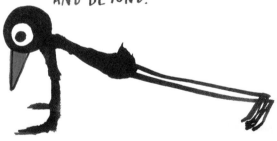

Strengthens
core and
spine

CoBRA

Bhuyangasana

LAY TUMMY DOWN,
PALMS ON FLOOR
UNDER SHOULDERS. PRESS
INTO HANDS TO LIFT UPPER
BODY, SLOWLY, OVER TIME.
BREATHE INTO LOWER BACK,
FEEL SPINE LENGTHENING.

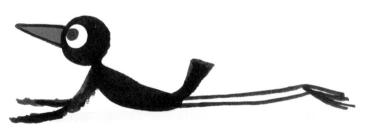

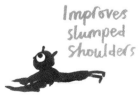

Improves
slumped
shoulders

UPWARD SALUTE

Urdhva Hastasana

FEET HIP-WIDTH APART,
INHALE, REACH UP YOUR
ARMS TO THE SKY.

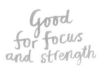

*Good
for focus
and strength*

HAPPY BABY

Ananda Balasana

LIE ON YOUR BACK
AND BEND KNEES
TO CHEST. HOLD
OUTSIDE OF ANKLES
OR FEET. ROCK GENTLY.

LOVE THIS POSE

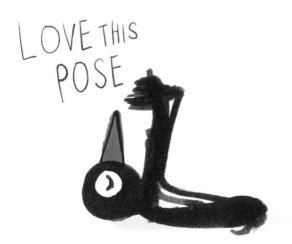

I'LL BE LAUGHED AT

Don't compare
yourself to
anyone

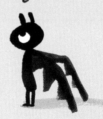

DOWNWARD-FACING DOG

Adho Mukha Svanasana

START ON ALL FOURS, HANDS SHOULDER-WIDTH APART. TUCK YOUR TOES, LIFT YOUR KNEES AND REACH HIPS UP AND BACK. BEND AND EXTEND LEGS TO RELEASE TENSION.

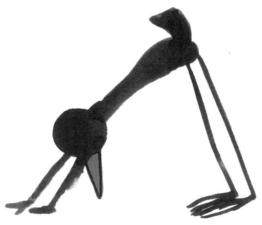

good for back pain

FOUR-LIMBED STAFF

Chaturanga Dandasana

FROM LYING, HANDS UNDER
SHOULDERS, ELBOWS DRAWN
BACK, TOES TUCKED, PRESS
DOWN TO LIFT BODY.

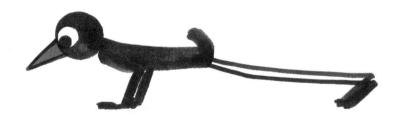

ONE-LEGGED DOWNWARD DOG

Eka Pada Adho Mukha Svanasana

FROM DOWNWARD DOG, ON THE INHALE, RAISE LEG IN LINE WITH THE BODY. PRESS HANDS ONTO FLOOR TO LIFT UP AND BACK THROUGH THE BODY TO THE FOOT.

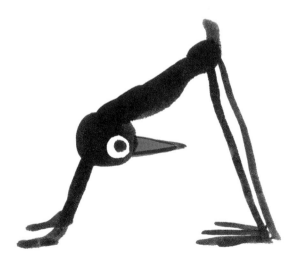

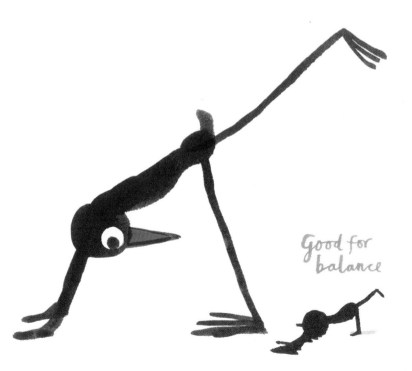

Good for
balance

SEATED FORWARD FOLD

Paschimottanasana

EXHALE, HINGE FROM
THE HIPS, FOLD FORWARD,
TOUCHING LEGS OR FEET.

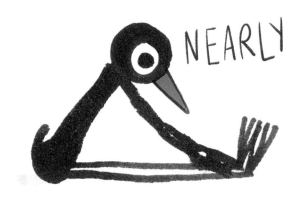

NEARLY

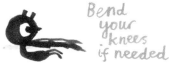

Bend
your
knees
if needed

STANDING FORWARD FOLD

Uttanasana

EXHALE, HINGE FROM THE HIPS, TOUCHING LEGS OR FEET.

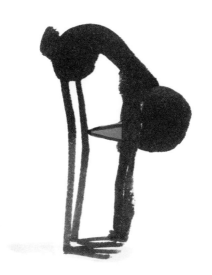

Has a calming effect

I CAN'T DO THIS

Be kind,
accept what
you can do

WARRIOR 1

Virabhadrasana 1

FEET HIP-WIDTH APART,
HIPS FACING FORWARD,
STEP YOUR RIGHT FOOT
FORWARD, BENDING YOUR
KNEE. STRETCH ARMS UP,
REACH TO THE SKY.

Good for balance

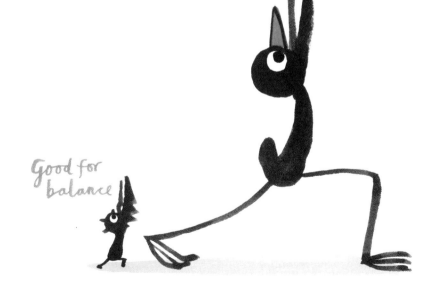

WARRIOR II

Virabhadrasana II

FEET WIDE AND PARALLEL,
TURN LEFT TOES IN 45°,
RIGHT TOES OUT 90°,
LUNGE TO RIGHT,
KNEE ABOVE ANKLE.
ARMS STRETCHED OUT
TO SIDE. REPEAT ON
OTHER SIDE.

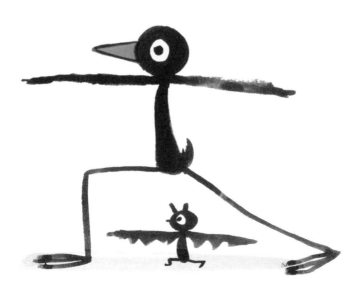

WARRIOR III

Virabhadrasana III

FOLD FORWARD FROM
HIPS. KEEPING LEFT FOOT
AND LEG STRONG, LIFT
RIGHT FOOT OFF FLOOR
SO THAT LEG AND TORSO
ARE PARALLEL TO FLOOR.
REVERSE ON OTHER SIDE.

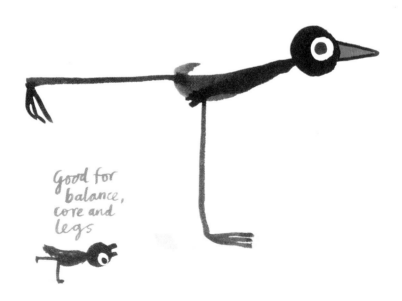

Good for
balance,
core and
legs

REVERSE WARRIOR

Viparita Virabhadrasana

FROM WARRIOR II, LIFT LEFT
ARM UP, RIGHT HAND ON
RIGHT THIGH. BREATHE INTO
LEFT SIDE OF BODY.

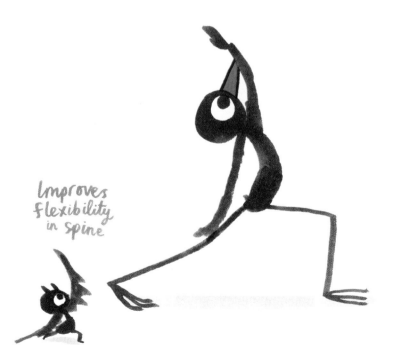

Improves
flexibility
in spine

SIMPLE FLOW SEQUENCE

1.

2.

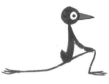

3.

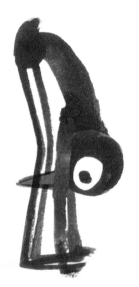

STANDING
1. FORWARD FOLD

Uttanasana

ON EXHALE, BEND
FROM HIPS, TOUCHING
LEGS OR TOES.

Has a
calming
effect

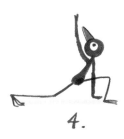

4.

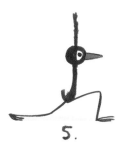

5.

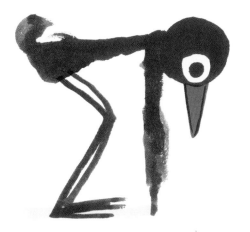

2. HALF STANDING FORWARD FOLD

Ardha Uttanasana

ON INHALE, LIFT HALFWAY UP, BACK FLAT.

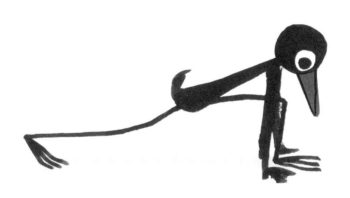

3. <u>LOW LUNGE</u>
Anjaneyasana

MOVE INTO LOW LUNGE,
RIGHT LEG STRETCHED
BACK, LEFT KNEE BENT.

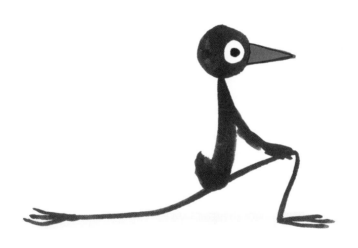

PLACE HANDS TO FRONT
KNEE OR FLOOR.
DROP BACK KNEE.

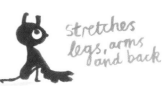

stretches
legs, arms
and back

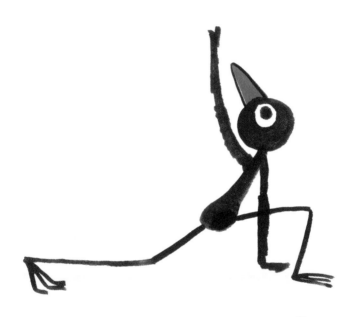

4. REVOLVED LUNGE

Parivrtta Utthita Ashwa
Sanchalanasana

RAISE RIGHT ARM.
LOOK UP, IF NECK
COMFORTABLE.

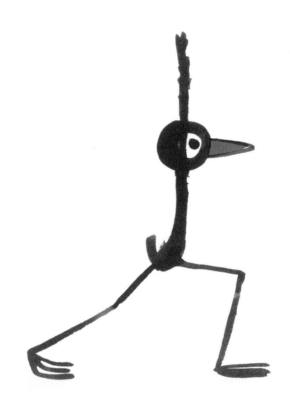

5. CRESCENT LUNGE

Ashta Chandrasana

FRONT KNEE ABOVE
ANKLE. BACK LEG
STRAIGHT AS POSSIBLE.
LIFT ARMS, PALMS FACING.

Strengthens
thighs, hips
and bottom

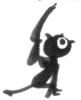

CHAIR
Utkatasana

BEND KNEES AND IMAGINE LIGHTLY
SITTING ON A CHAIR, TAILBONE DOWN.
RAISE ARMS TO THE SKY. FOCUS YOUR
GAZE A FEW FEET AHEAD ON FLOOR.

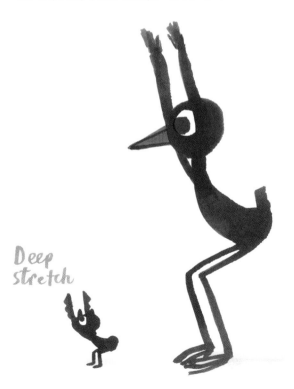

Deep
stretch

TRY USING A WALL
TO SUPPORT YOUR BACK.

HARDER THAN
IT LOOKS

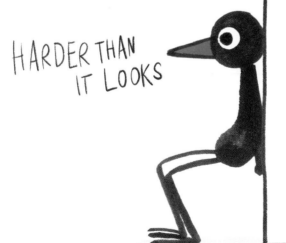

I
DON'T
HAVE
TIME

Start
with 5
minutes
a day

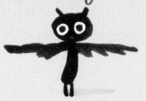

SEATED POSE

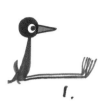 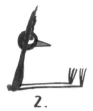 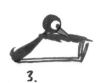

1.   2.   3.

<u>STAFF</u> MOVING TO <u>SEATED FORWARD FOLD.</u>

<u>STAFF</u>
Dandasana

1. **SIT DOWN** (YOU CAN SIT ON A FOLDED BLANKET), **LEGS STRAIGHT, PALMS DRAWING DOWN.**

Relax
Shoulders
and face

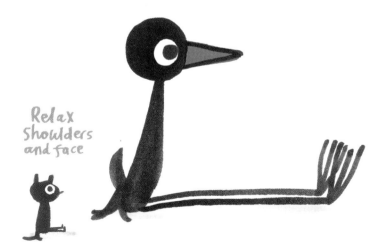

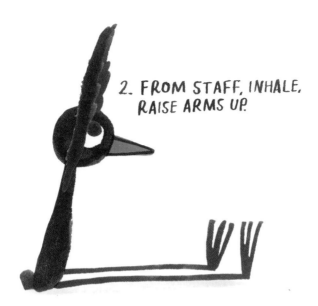

2. FROM STAFF, INHALE, RAISE ARMS UP.

SEATED FORWARD FOLD

Paschimottanasana

3. EXHALE, FOLD FORWARD FROM HIPS, HANDS TO LEGS OR FEET.

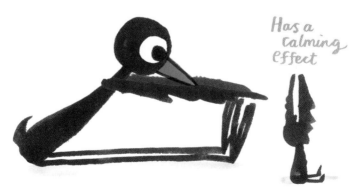

Has a calming effect

DOLPHIN

Ardha Pincha Mayurasana

START ON ALL FOURS,
BEND ELBOWS TO FLOOR.
LIFT HIPS TO SKY, TOES
TUCKED. BEND KNEES
TO RELEASE HAMSTRINGS.

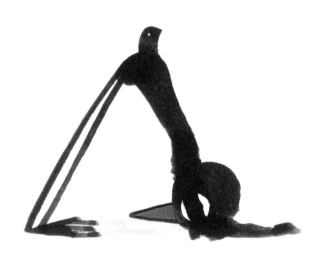

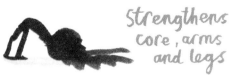

Strengthens
core, arms
and legs

EXTENDED PUPPY

Uttana Shishosana

FROM ALL FOURS,
WALK HANDS FORWARD
AS YOU RAISE YOUR HIPS.
LET YOUR CHEST MELT
DOWNWARD AND REST
FOREHEAD ON THE FLOOR.

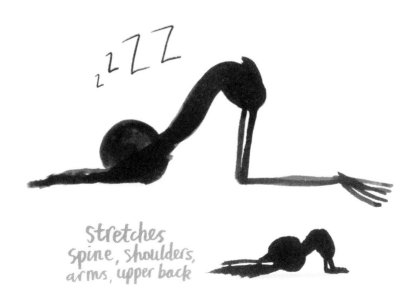

Stretches
spine, shoulders,
arms, upper back

TRIANGLE

Utthita Trikonasana

LEGS WIDE, FEET TURNED AS
IN WARRIOR II. HINGE FROM
HIPS, EXTENDING RIBS TO RIGHT.
LET RIGHT HAND DROP TO LEG
OR FLOOR, RIGHT ARM UP.
REPEAT ON OTHER SIDE.

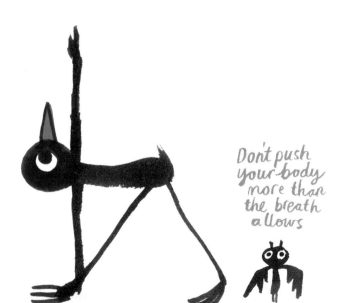

Don't push
your body
more than
the breath
allows

CHILD
Balasana

KNEEL WITH KNEES
WIDE, BIG TOES TOGETHER.
LEAN TORSO FORWARDS,
KEEPING SITTING BONES
DOWN IF POSSIBLE.
STRETCH ARMS IN FRONT
OR BY SIDE OF BODY.

I RECOVER
HERE

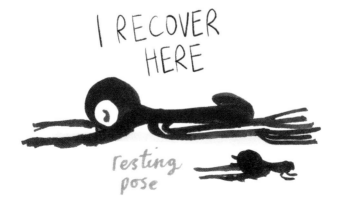

resting
pose

SUN SALUTATION A

Surya Namaskar A

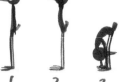

1.   2.   3.   4.   5.   6.

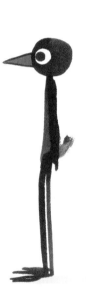 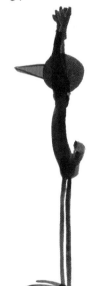 

1. MOUNTAIN

Tadasana

STAND UPRIGHT, FEET
HIP-WIDTH APART.

2. UPWARD SALUTE

Urdhva Hastasana

INHALE, REACH UP YOUR
HANDS TO THE SKY.

THE SUN SALUTATION IS A SEQUENCE (VINYASA) OF YOGA POSES (ASANAS). IT'S A GREAT WAY TO BEGIN YOUR DAY, BRINGING GRATITUDE TO THE SUN FOR ITS ENERGY (PRANA).

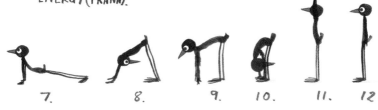

7.   8.   9.   10.   11.   12.

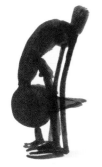

3. STANDING FORWARD FOLD

Uttanasana

EXHALE, BEND OVER, TOUCHING LEGS OR FEET.

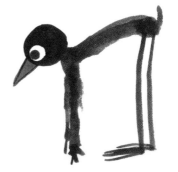

4. HALF STANDING FORWARD FOLD

Ardha Uttanasana

INHALE, LIFT HALFWAY UP, BACK FLAT.

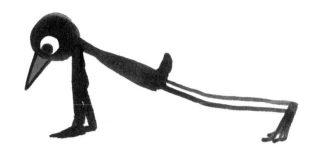

5. HIGH PLANK

Kumbhakasana

EXHALE, STEP BACK TO
HIGH PLANK. DROP KNEES
IF NEEDED.

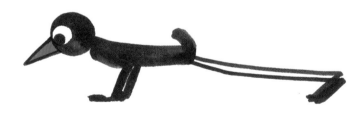

6. PLANK

Chaturanga Dandasana

EXHALE, BEND
ELBOWS BACK AND
DRAW IN TO BODY.

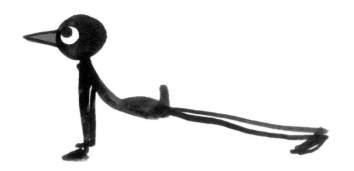

7. <u>UPWARD-FACING DOG</u>

Urdhwa Mukha Svanasana

INHALE, STRAIGHTEN ARMS,
HEART LIFTING, ROLL UP
THROUGH SPINE.

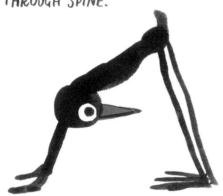

8. <u>DOWNWARD-FACING DOG</u>

Adho Mukha Svanasana

EXHALE, HIPS UP AND BACK.
BEND KNEES TO RELEASE
HAMSTRINGS.

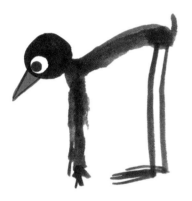

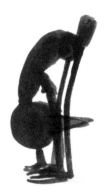

9. HALF STANDING FORWARD FOLD

Ardha Uttanasana

INHALE AS YOU STEP OR JUMP BACK TO HANDS. HANDS TO LEGS OR FLOOR, LIFT HALFWAY UP.

10. STANDING FORWARD FOLD

Uttanasana

EXHALE, FOLD OVER, TOUCHING LEGS OR FEET.

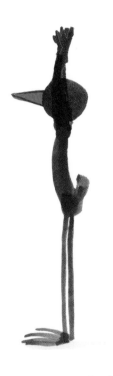

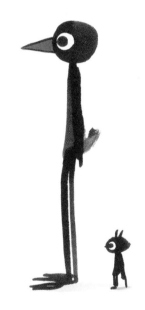

11. UPWARD SALUTE

Urdhva Hastasana

INHALE, REACH UP YOUR
HANDS TO THE SKY.

12. MOUNTAIN

Tadasana

BACK TO STANDING.
GROUND THROUGH FEET.

I DON'T BEND that WAY

A calm
mind is
more
important
than a
bendy body

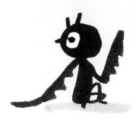

BRIDGE

Setu Bandha Sarvangasana

LIE ON YOUR BACK, KNEES
BENT, HIP-DISTANCE APART.
PRESS DOWN THROUGH FEET,
INHALE, AND LIFT HIPS. CLASP
HANDS UNDER LOWER BACK
AND LIFT HIGHER, ROLLING
SHOULDER BLADES TOWARDS SPINE.
PRESS FEET AND HANDS TO FLOOR.
EXHALE TO SLOWLY ROLL BACK DOWN.

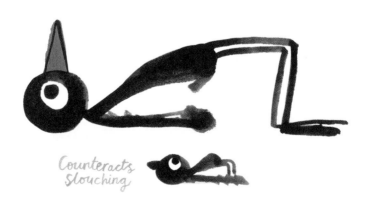

Counteracts
Slouching

FISH

Matsyasana

LIE ON YOUR BACK, BEND
KNEES. LIFT HIPS AND
SLIDE HANDS UNDER BOTTOM.
INHALE, EXTEND LEGS. LIFT AND
OPEN CHEST. PRESS INTO ELBOWS.
DON'T STRAIN YOUR NECK, USE A
SUPPORT FOR HEAD IF NEEDED.

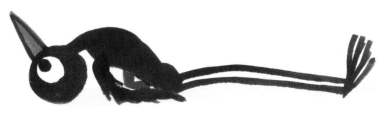

Relieves
tension
in neck
and throat

GARLAND

Malasana

TURN LEGS OUT FROM
HIPS. SQUAT DOWN
SLOWLY. SPINE LONG,
CHEST OPEN, GAZE
FORWARD. PALMS
TOGETHER AT CHEST.

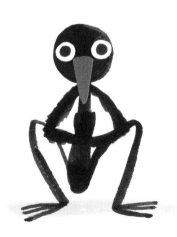

RAISE HEELS OR
REST ON SUPPORT
IF NEEDED.

Good for
pelvic floor
and digestion

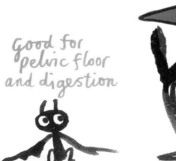

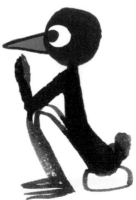

I AM
A TREE

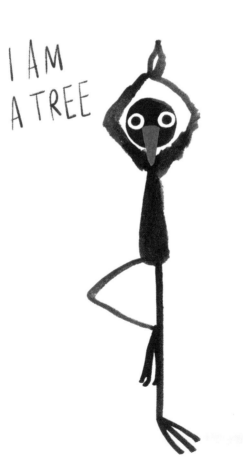

TREE

Vrksasana

PLACE FOOT ON
INSIDE OF STANDING
LEG, HIGH OR LOW.
HANDS WITH PALMS
TOGETHER AT CHEST
OR RAISED TO SKY.
BREATHE!

Good for
balance

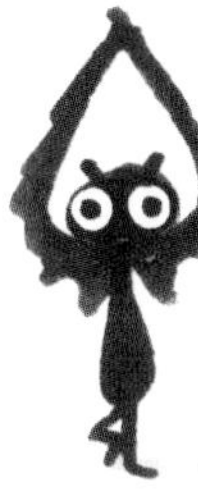

YOGA SEQUENCE FOR ENERGY

Try and hold each pose for 5-10 breaths.

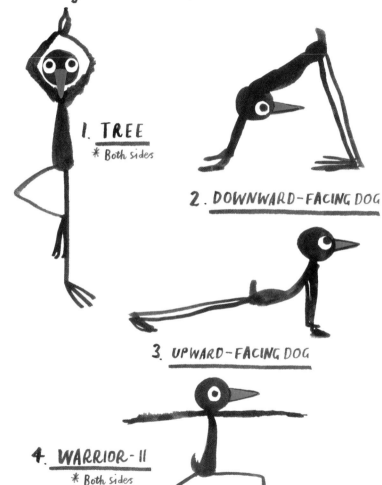

1. TREE
* Both sides

2. DOWNWARD-FACING DOG

3. UPWARD-FACING DOG

4. WARRIOR-II
* Both sides

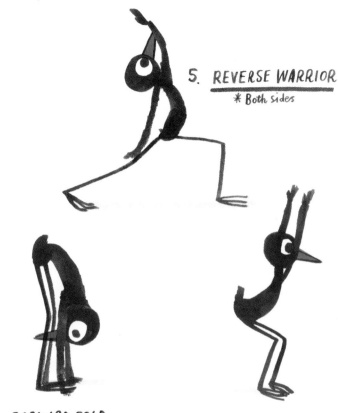

5. REVERSE WARRIOR
* Both sides

6. FORWARD FOLD

7. CHAIR

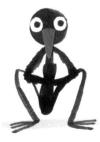

8. GARLAND

MY MIND KEEPS WANDERING

Come
back
to the
BREATH

TWISTY

EAGLE

Garudasana

FROM CHAIR POSE
CROSS LEFT LEG OVER
RIGHT THIGH. CROSS
ARMS, RIGHT OVER LEFT
IN AN 'X', THEN BEND ELBOWS,
WINDING LEFT ARM IN
TOWARDS RIGHT, HANDS
MOVING CLOSER.
REPEAT OTHER SIDE.

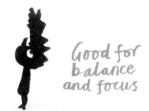

Good for
balance
and focus

BACK ARCH

PIGEON

Eka Pada Rajakapotasana

FROM ALL FOURS,
SLIDE LEFT KNEE
BEYOND LEFT WRIST,
TAKE LEFT FOOT TOWARDS
RIGHT WRIST. EASE
RIGHT LEG BACK,
HIPS SQUARED.
REPEAT OTHER SIDE.

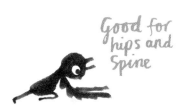

Good for
hips and
spine

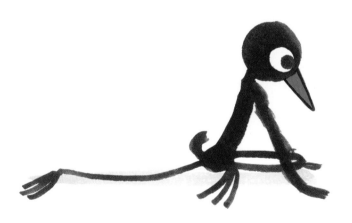

HALF LORD OF THE FISHES

Ardha Matsyendrasana

FROM STAFF POSE,
STEP RIGHT FOOT OVER
LEFT THIGH. BRING
LEFT FOOT TO THE
OUTSIDE OF RIGHT HIP.
ON EXHALE, TWIST BODY
GENTLY TO THE RIGHT.
RIGHT ARM BEHIND
YOU, LEFT ARM HUGS
LEFT KNEE.
REPEAT ON OTHER SIDE.

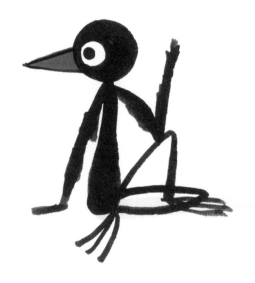

Good for
posture
and digestion

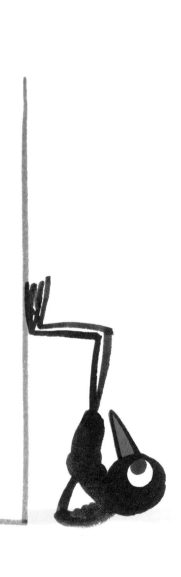

SUPPORTED SHOULDERSTAND
Salamba Sarvangasana

A GENTLE OPTION FOR A SHOULDERSTAND IS TO PRESS YOUR FEET INTO A WALL AND LIFT PELVIS OFF THE FLOOR. SUPPORT HIPS WITH HANDS. NECK SHOULD FEEL COMFORTABLE.

THIS IS A GOOD PREPARATION FOR PLOUGH.

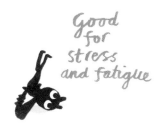

Good for stress and fatigue

PLOUGH
Halasana

FROM LYING, PRESS ARMS
AND HANDS INTO GROUND
TO ROLL KNEES TO CHEST,
LIFTING HIPS. SUPPORT
BACK WITH HANDS. EXTEND
LEGS ONCE SPINE LIFTED.
KEEPING SPINE LIFTED,
RELEASE ARMS AND HANDS
TO FLOOR, PALMS DOWN.

TO RELEASE, ROLL DOWN
SLOWLY, ONE VERTEBRA
AT A TIME.

I CAN ONLY
DO THIS IN
MY DREAMS.

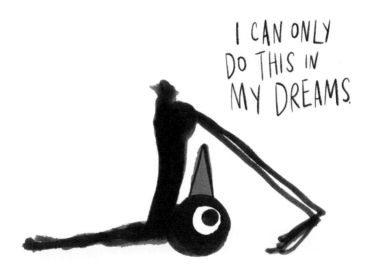

me
too

I'M
NOT
GOOD
ENOUGH

Be
better
than
yesterday

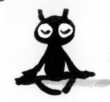

LOCUST
Salabhasana

LIE ON TUMMY,
SLOWLY LIFT AND
EXTEND CHEST, HEAD
AND LEGS FROM THE
FLOOR. REACH ARMS
BACK, ROLLING
SHOULDERS IN, PALMS
TURNED TO BODY.

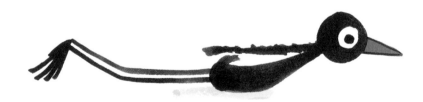

Opens
chest and
Shoulders

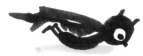

HERO

Virasana

KNEEL, KNEES TOGETHER,
FEET APART, BOTTOM
ON FLOOR OR PILLOWS.
ALLOW SPINE TO LIFT.
REST HANDS ON LAP.

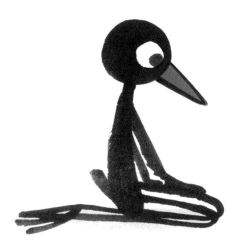

A good
alternative
to sitting
cross-legged

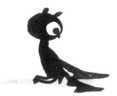

CORPSE
Savasana

CORPSE POSE IS
THE MOST IMPORTANT
POSTURE! ALWAYS LIE
DOWN AT THE END OF
YOUR PRACTICE.
BREATHE. BE COMPLETELY
IN THE MOMENT.

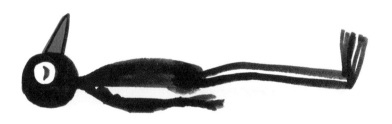

My favourite
yoga pose

YOGA POSES FOR BEDTIME

Try and hold each pose for 5-10 breaths.

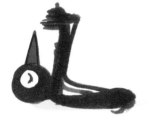

1. HAPPY BABY

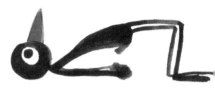

2. BRIDGE

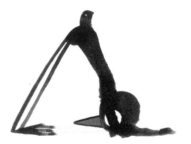

3. DOLPHIN

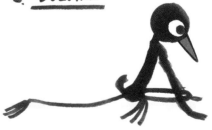

4. PIGEON

* Both sides

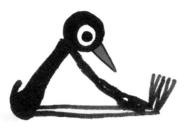

5. SEATED FORWARD FOLD

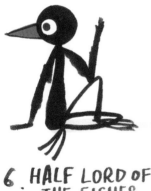

6. HALF LORD OF THE FISHES

* Both sides

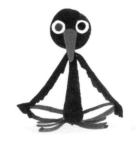

7. EASY/COMFORTABLE

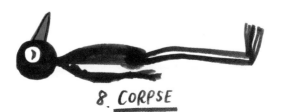

8. CORPSE

Come to
this pose
any time
you need to

MARION WOULD LIKE TO THANK ZARA LARCOMBE,
ROLY ALLEN, GAYNOR SERMON, FELICITY AWDRY,
LEONIE TAYLOR; VANESSA GREEN AT THE URBAN ANT,
ANGUS HYLAND, AND ELIZABETH SHEINKMAN PFD.
PROUD TO BE PART OF THE FIRST SEASON OF
SKITTLEDOG BOOKS.

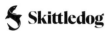 **Skittledog**

FIRST PUBLISHED IN THE UNITED KINGDOM IN 2023
BY SKITTLEDOG, AN IMPRINT OF THAMES & HUDSON LTD,
181A HIGH HOLBORN, LONDON WC1V 7QX

REPRINTED 2023

BRITISH LIBRARY CATALOGUING-IN-PUBLICATION DATA
A CATALOGUE RECORD FOR THIS BOOK IS AVAILABLE FROM
THE BRITISH LIBRARY

ISBN 978-1-837-76012-1

PRINTED AND BOUND IN ITALY BY LEGO SPA

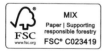

BE THE FIRST TO KNOW ABOUT OUR NEW RELEASES,
EXCLUSIVE CONTENT AND AUTHOR EVENTS BY VISITING
SKITTLEDOG.COM
THAMESANDHUDSON.COM